Exercises
For
Therapeutic Riding

Exercises for Therapeutic Riding

By

Jerri Lincoln

Photographs by
Lisa Hollenbeck

Ralston Store Publishing
P.O. Box 4513
Durango, Colorado 81302

ISBN 978-0-9822585-7-6

Disclaimer of Liability:
Not all exercise is suitable for everyone, and this or any exercise program may result in injury. Please seek a physician's advice before beginning any new exercise program. The author and publisher assume no responsibility for injuries suffered while practicing these techniques.

Printed in the USA

It is always a debate over who gets more from therapeutic riding: the clients or the volunteers. As a volunteer, I feel certain that I do.

This book contains a broad array of exercises. Some are simple, some are more complex. Some require more balance than others. All exercises should be monitored, and some exercises will require assistance. And of course, before starting, all exercises should be evaluated for horse and rider.

These exercises should not feel painful. Gradual repetition achieves results.

This book is dedicated to all therapeutic riding horses, without whose patience and love therapeutic riding would not be possible.

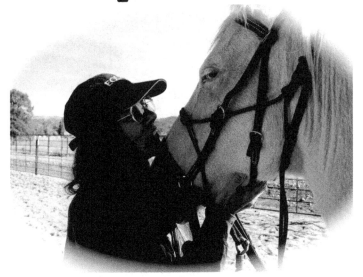

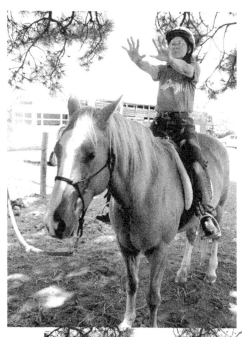

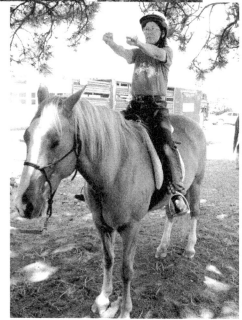

Extend both arms straight out in front of you. Stretch out and reach with your fingers as you inhale. As you exhale, clench your fingers into a fist. Repeat this pose four more times while continuing to inhale and exhale. This pose strengthens the finger and hand muscles.

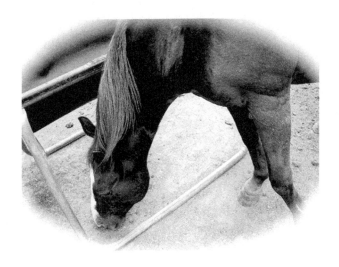

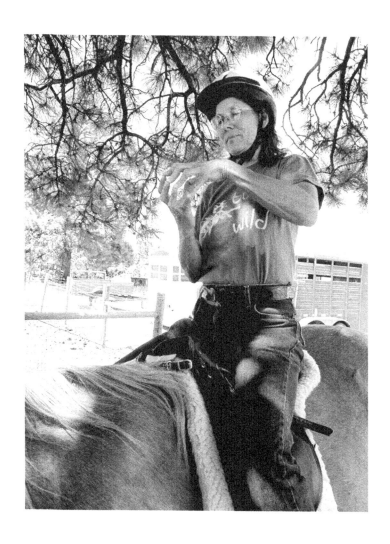

Place your fingertips together
exerting some pressure. Now, like
a spider doing push ups on a
mirror, push your fingers against
each other so the palms of your
hand come closer together and
then farther apart. Continue while
exerting pressure. This pose
strengthens the finger and hand
muscles.

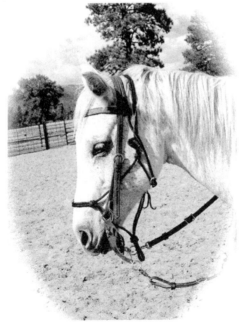

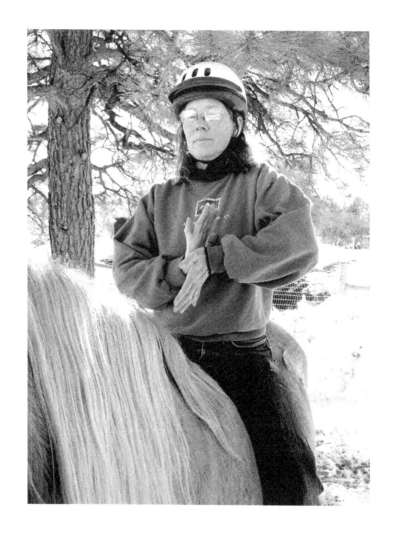

With equal pressure, press the heel of one palm against the heel of the other palm. Take one complete slow breath. First, have one hand facing up, and then the other hand. Continue breathing, and do each hand three times. This pose tightens the hand muscles.

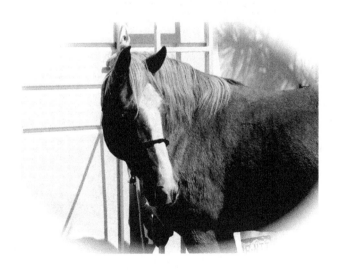

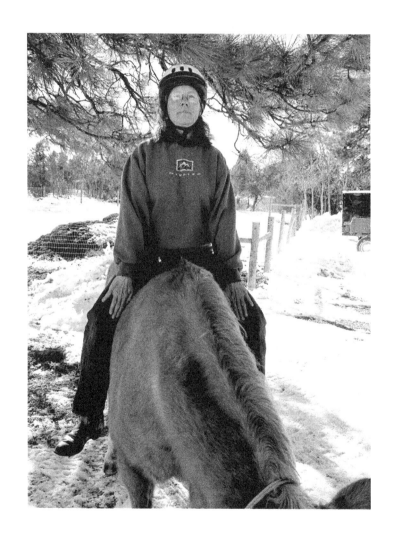

Place your hands on the inside of your thighs, just behind the knees. Inhale as you try to press your thighs together while pushing outward with your hands. Exhale and relax. Repeat four times. This pose strengthens the thighs, and the upper arms.

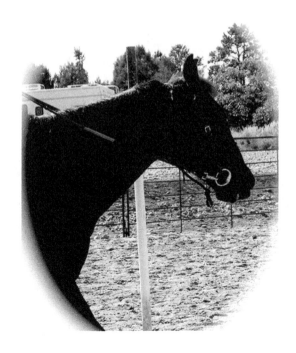

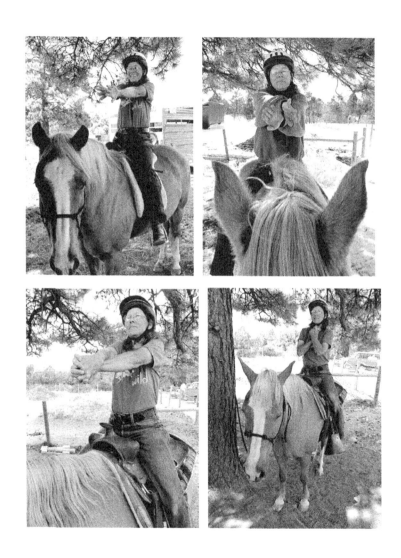

Hold your arms straight out in front of you, with your palms facing outward. Cross the right hand over the left hand. Your palms should now face each other. Interlace your fingers. Inhale as you pull your hands toward your stomach, and then up toward your chin keeping the fingers interlaced. Exhale as you stretch your arms back out, keeping the fingers interlaced. Repeat this three times remembering to inhale and exhale! Then, start again with your arms straight out in front, and this time do the entire exercise with your left hand crossed over your right hand. Repeat three times. This pose strengthens the arm muscles, calms the mind, and improves concentration.

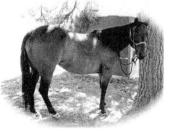

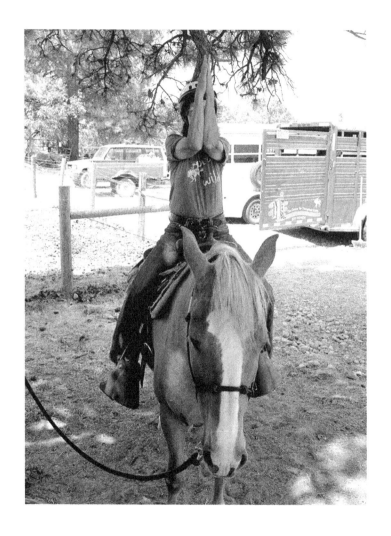

Extend your arms straight out in front of you, with the palms together and the elbows together. Keeping hands and elbows pressed together, bend at the elbow and bring your hands toward your forehead, until they are at a ninety-degree angle. Raise your arms upward as far as is comfortable. Hold the pose for five deep breaths. This pose strengthens and aligns the upper body.

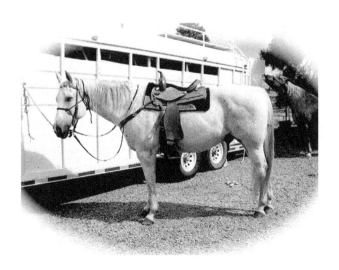

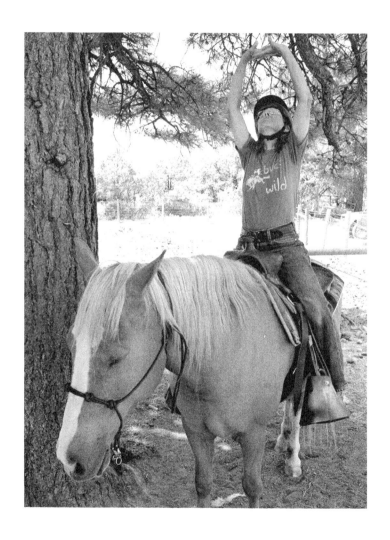

With your back straight, inhale and raise your arms over your head with your palms together. Interlace your fingers and press your palms away from your body stretching your arms and your spine upward. Tilt your head back gently to look at your hands. Exhale and take four more deep breaths. This pose stretches the belly, improves digestion, and increases circulation to the upper body and the arms, hands, and wrists.

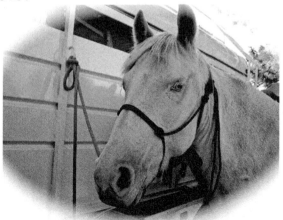

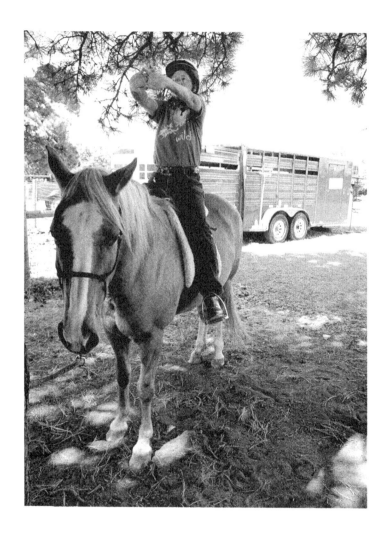

Interlace your fingers and press your palms away from your body keeping your arms at shoulder level. Hold the pose as you take five deep breaths. This pose stretches the shoulders, upper arms, and forearms.

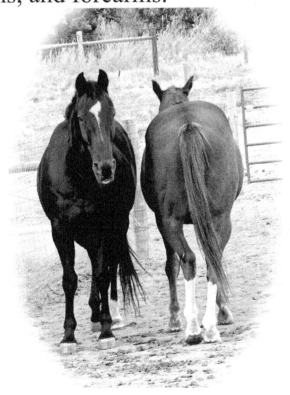

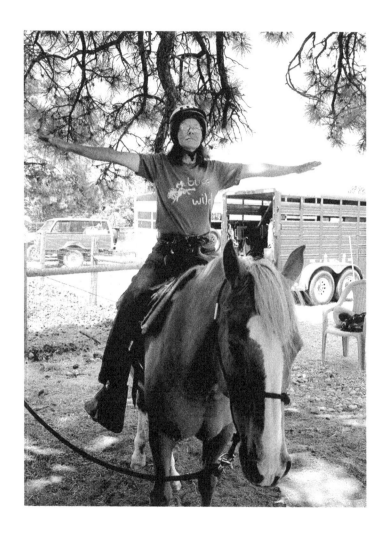

Stretch both arms out to the side at shoulder level. Feel the stretch from your shoulders and upper back to the tips of your fingers.

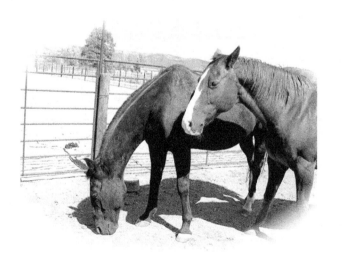

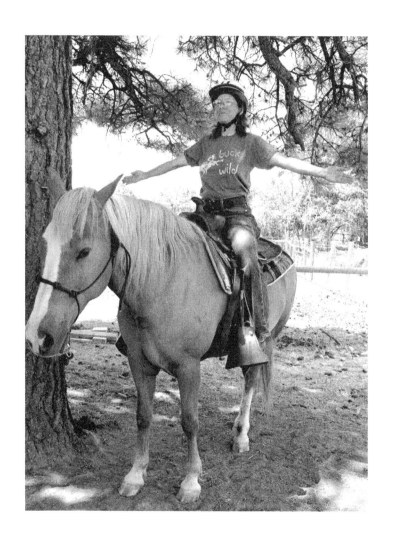

Rotate your arms forward ten times in large circles. Reverse direction for ten more times. This pose strengthens the shoulders and upper arms.

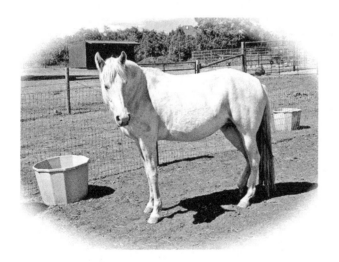

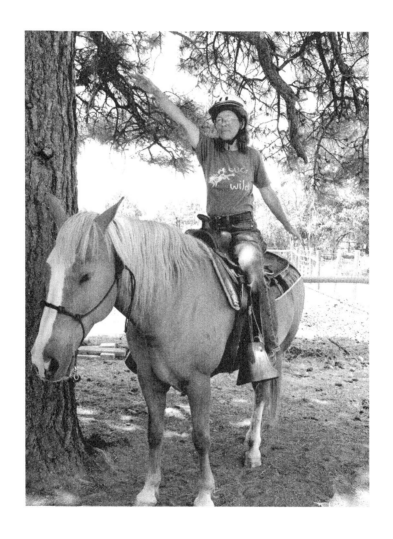

"Swim" with the crawl stroke ten times for each arm. Then reverse, and do the "back stroke" ten times for each arm. This exercise is good for your arms and upper body.

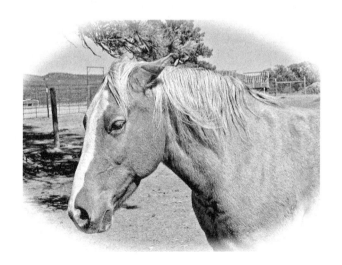

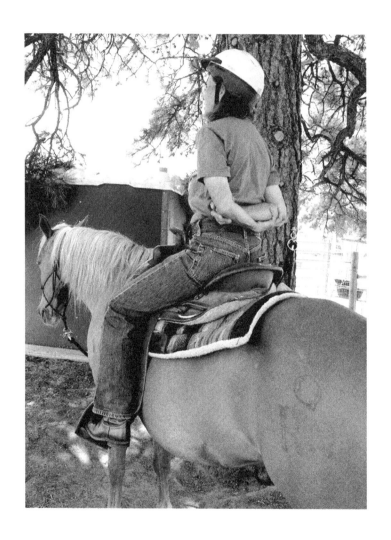

Put both hands behind your back, and clasp your arms as close as you can to the elbows. Breathe five deep breaths. Now put the opposite arm on top, and breathe five more deep breaths. This pose stretches the muscles and tendons of the arms and upper chest.

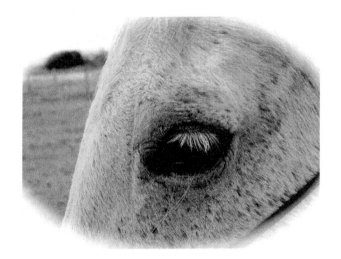

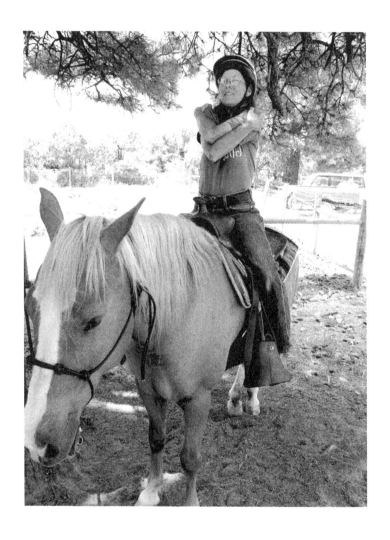

Wrap your arms around yourself
in a big hug. But, not so tight that
you can't breathe! Take five deep
breaths. Notice which arm is on
top, and switch arms. Take five
more deep breaths. This pose
stretches the arms, and feels really
good!

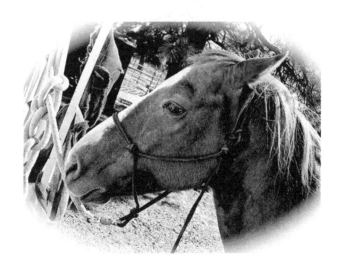

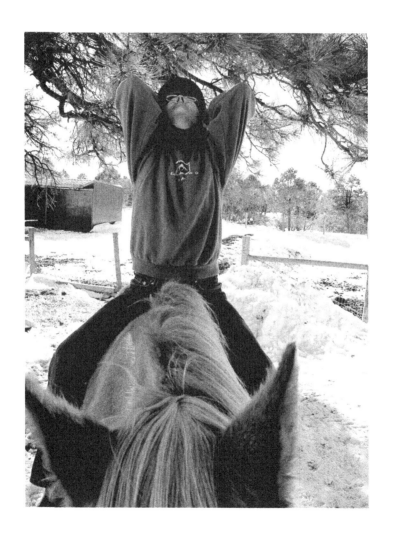

Reach behind you as if you are reaching for the back of a chair, right hand over right shoulder, and left hand over left shoulder. Your head goes back gently stretching your neck and you should have a slight arch to your back. Breathe deeply for five breaths. This pose increases flexibility in the back.

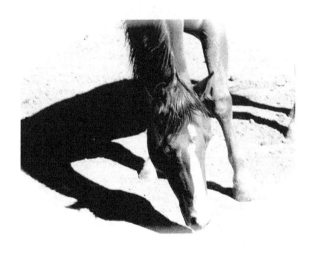

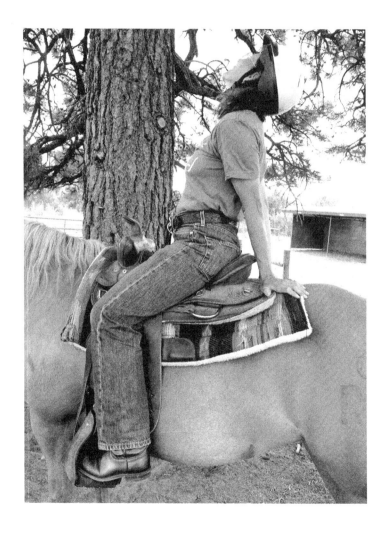

Place your hands behind you on the saddle or the horse. Inhale and lift your chest upward as you look upward. Continue breathing five deep breaths. This pose increases flexibility in the back and shoulders.

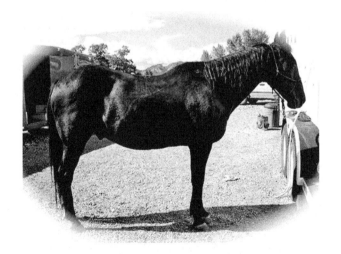

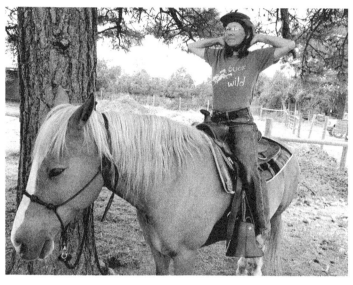

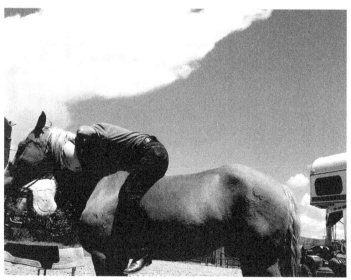

Put your hands gently behind your head, fingers barely touching, not pushing on your head. Come forward slowly into a forward bend, without putting any pressure on your head. Breathe five deep breaths, and then come up slowly one vertebra at a time. This pose stretches the arms, the hips, and the back.

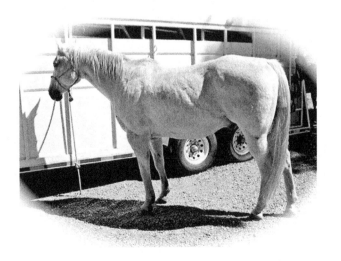

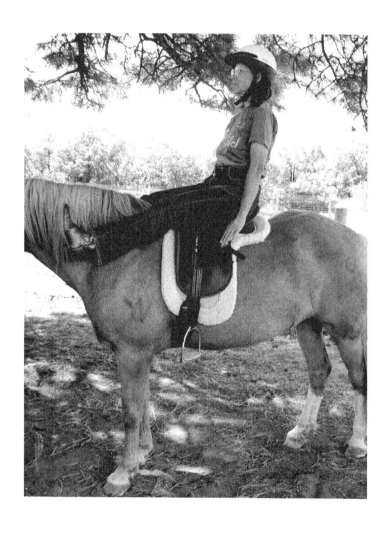

Stretch your right leg out in front of you. Do not lock the knee; keep a slight bend in it. Hold it there for five slow, deep breaths. Gently lower it, and stretch the left leg out in front of you, without locking the knee. Hold it there for five slow, deep breaths. This pose strengthens your legs, lower back muscles, and abdominal area.

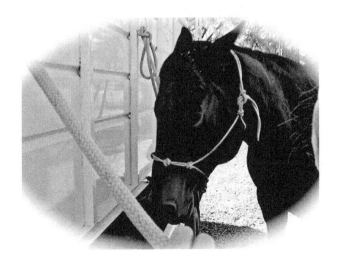

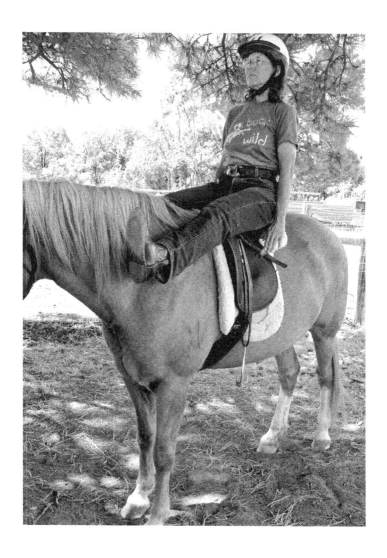

Stretch both legs out in front of you without locking the knees. Hold them there for five slow, deep breaths before you gently lower them to the ground. This pose strengthens your legs, lower back muscles, and abdominal area.

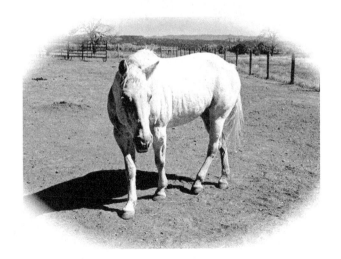

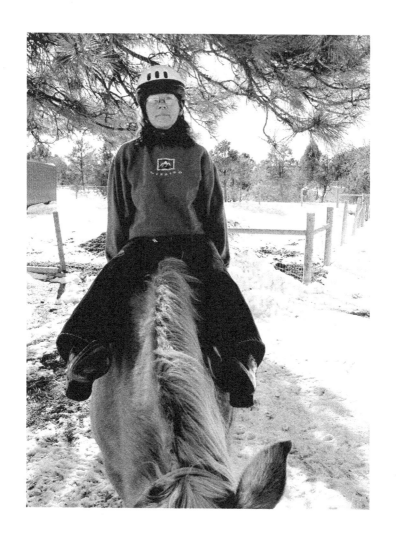

Stretch your legs straight out in front of you. Point and flex your feet. Then rotate your feet in place, first one direction and then the other. This pose loosens and lubricates the joints.

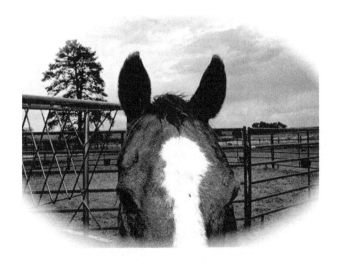

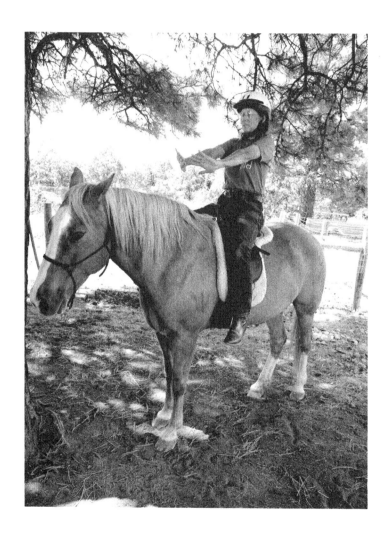

Stretch your arms straight out in front of you. Flex your wrists up and down, and then rotate them first in one direction and then the other. This pose loosens and lubricates the joints.

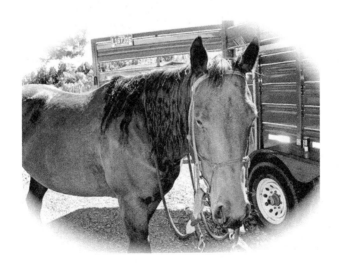

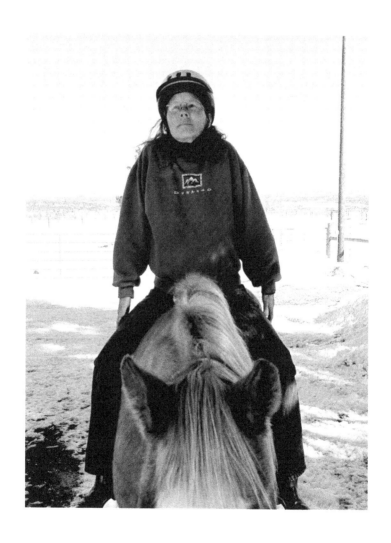

Sit up straight. Inhale as you raise your shoulders toward your ears. Exhale, and let them drop back down. Repeat five times. This pose strengthens the shoulder area, and relieves tension in the neck and shoulders.

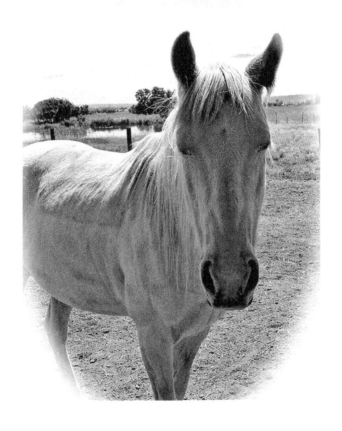

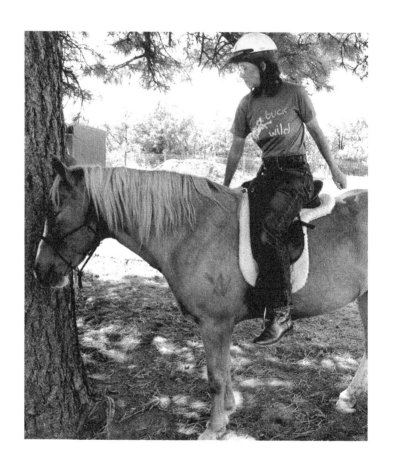

With your back straight, and looking straight ahead, roll one shoulder forward and then the other, like walking with your shoulders. Do each shoulder five times, and then reverse the direction by rolling each shoulder backwards five times, like walking backwards. This pose strengthens the shoulders, and relieves tension.

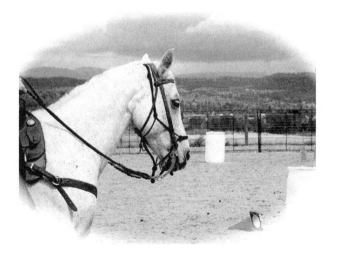

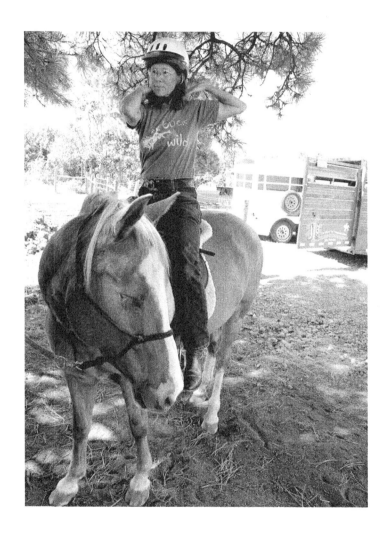

Place your right hand on your right shoulder, and your left hand on your left shoulder. Now begin making swimming-like movements, by moving your elbow forward and then around, first one elbow and then the other. Repeat five times, and then reverse direction by moving your elbow back and then around. Repeat five times. This pose strengthens the shoulders, and releases tension in the shoulder and upper back.

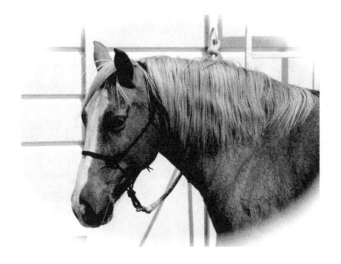

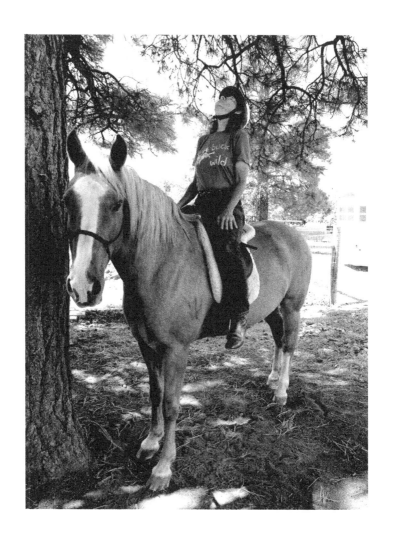

Take a deep breath. With your back straight, and looking straight ahead, on the exhale tilt your head forward so your chin goes toward your chest. Inhale back up. Repeat two more times. On the next exhale, lift your chin and tilt your head backward toward your back. Inhale back up, and repeat two more times. On the next exhale, bring your right ear toward your shoulder. Inhale back up, and repeat two more times. Next exhale, bring your left ear toward your shoulder. Inhale back up, and repeat two more times. Turn your head to look over each shoulder in turn. Finally, starting at the chin toward chest position, move your head toward the right, then the back, then the left, then the chest again, doing neck circles. Do the circle twice in each direction. This pose creates greater flexibility and range of motion in the neck.

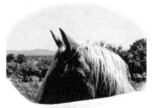

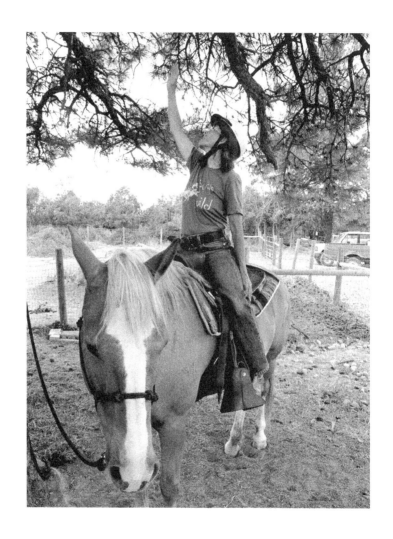

Keeping your back straight, inhale as you raise one arm over your head, turning your head to look up at it. Exhale and bring the arm back down. Inhale as you raise the other arm over your head, turning your head to look up at it. Exhale and bring the arm back down. Raise each arm four more times. This pose lengthens and strengthens the back, and strengthens the shoulders.

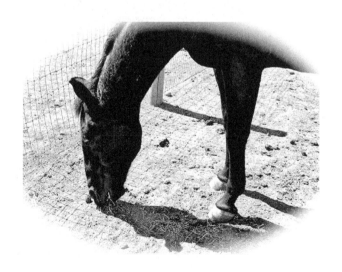

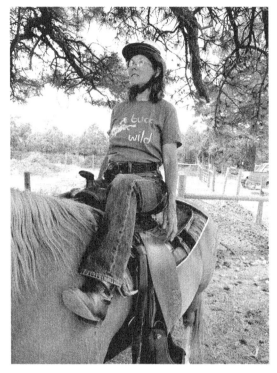

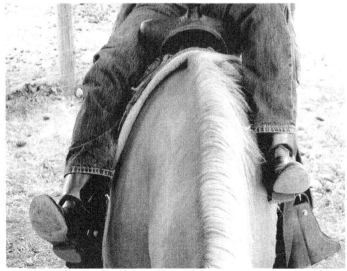

Raise your legs, and make pedaling movements as if you are riding a bicycle. Breathe deep and continue the cycling movements for five deep breaths. This pose strengthens the leg muscles.

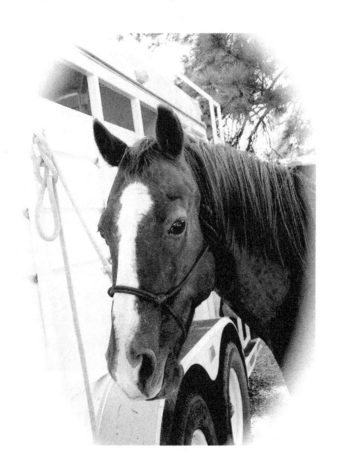

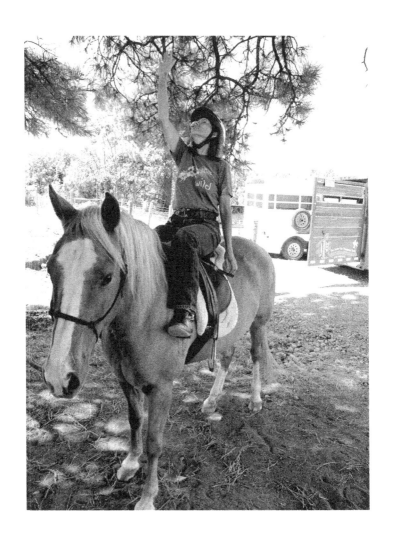

Slowly raise your left leg keeping your knee bent, and at the same time raise your right arm. As you lower them, slowly raise your right leg keeping your knee bent, and at the same time raise your left arm. Continue marching in place, and repeat ten times. This pose promotes balance between both hemispheres of the brain, as well as strengthening arms and legs.

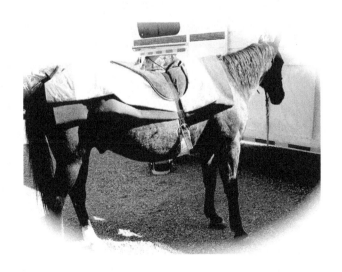

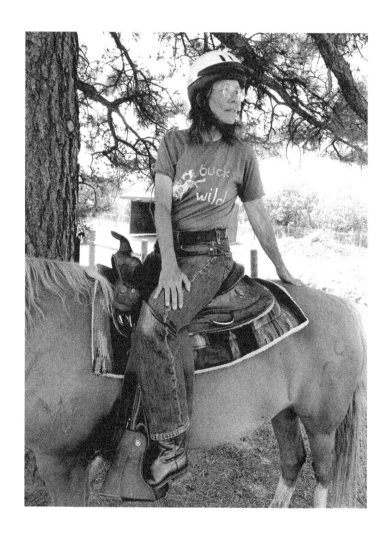

Put your left hand on your right
knee. With your knees facing
forward, turn your body to the
right and look right. Take five
deep breaths. Come slowly back
to center. Put your right hand on
your left knee. With your knees
still facing forward, turn your
body to the left and look left.
Take five more deep breaths. This
pose stretches the back, the
shoulders, and the hips.

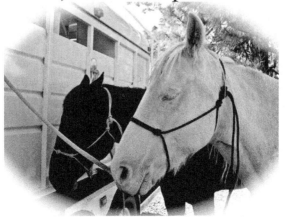

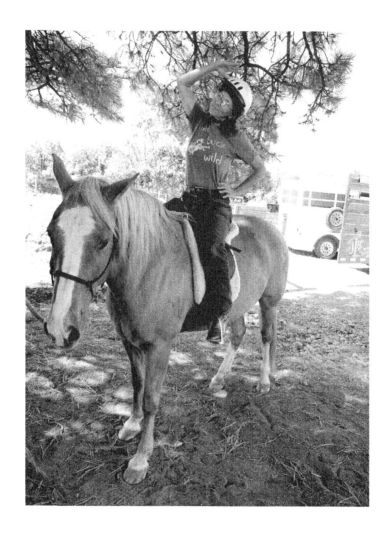

Raise your right arm straight up, and put your left hand on your left hip. Bend toward the left, bringing your right hand over your head. Hold for five breaths. Come back to center and lower your arm. Raise your left arm straight up, and put your right hand on your right hip. Bend toward the right, bringing your left hand over your head. Hold for five breaths. This pose strengthens the spine, the neck, and the arms.

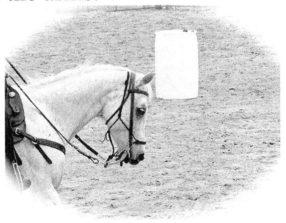

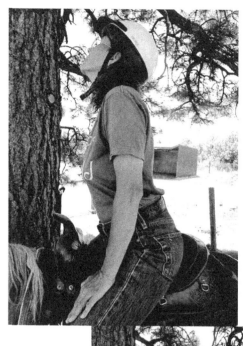

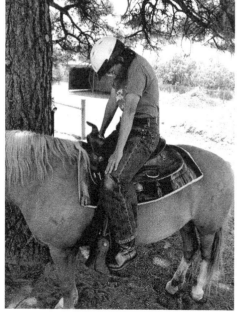

Start with your back straight and your hands on your knees. Slowly inhale and lift your chest up and forward, creating a slight arch in your back while your head faces forward and slightly up. Slowly exhale while rounding your back, pulling in your belly, and tucking your chin into your chest. Repeat this slowly five times. These two poses increase spinal flexibility and abdominal strength.

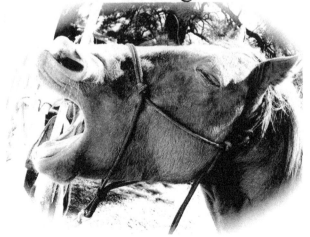

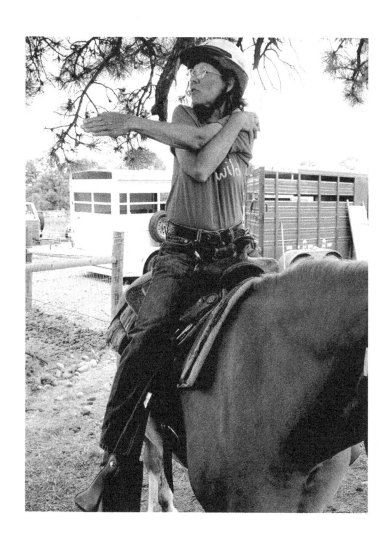

Reach straight out in front of you with your right arm, while stretching your fingers. Move your arm slowly to the left. Take your left hand and put it on your right upper arm, and pull it in toward your chest. Hold for five deep breaths. Release your right arm. Now, reach straight out in front of you with your left arm, while stretching your fingers. Move your arm slowly to the right. Take your right hand and put it on your left upper arm, and pull it in toward your chest. Hold for five deep breaths. This is a good stretch for your shoulders.

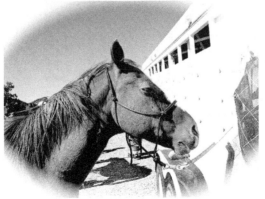

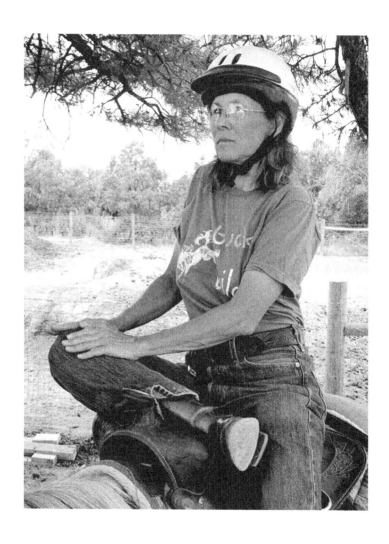

Place your right ankle over your left knee. Put your right hand on your knee and exhale as you gently push the knee downward. Inhale as you release pressure. Do this three times, and then put your left ankle over your right knee and exhale as you gently push the knee downward. Inhale as you release pressure. Do this three times. This pose is a good stretch for the hips.

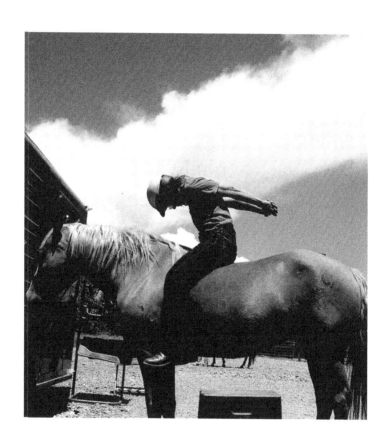

Reach both arms behind your back and interlace your fingers. Now lean forward and raise your arms as high as they will comfortably go. Take five slow deep breaths. This pose stretches the muscles in the chest and the shoulders.

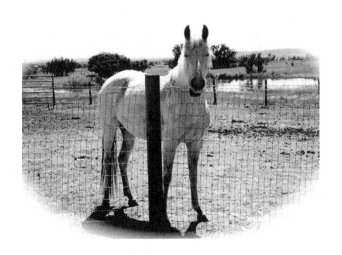

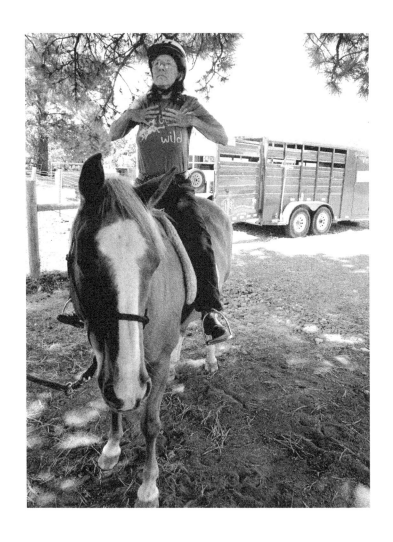

Put your thumbs in your armpits, and flap your arms energetically! This pose releases tension in the shoulders.

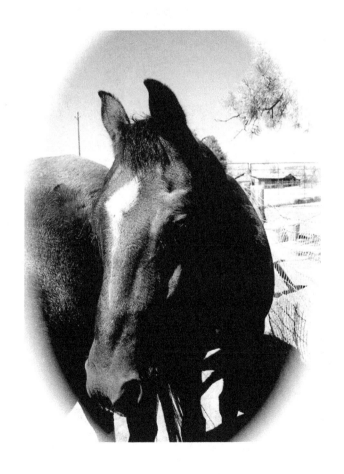

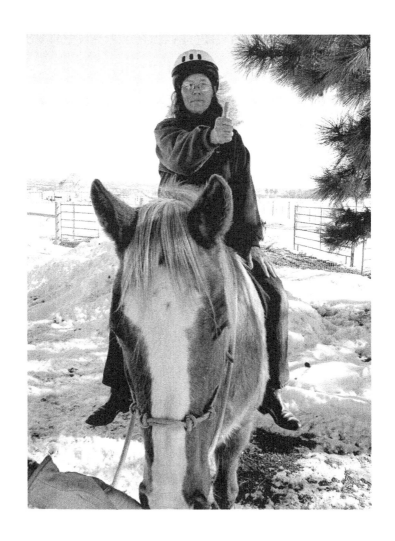

Reach out in front of you with your right hand, thumb up. Move it slightly left so it is in the center of your body. Start by moving your thumb up to the left, and draw sideways figure eights. Make sure that the thumb crosses the midline of your body. Keep going to make five figure eights, and then do the same thing five times with your left hand, moving up to the right. Follow your thumb with your eyes, but don't move your head. This pose balances the two hemispheres of the brain.

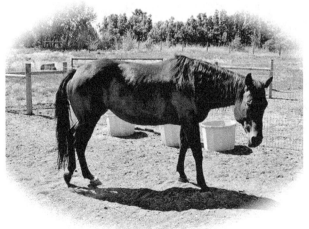

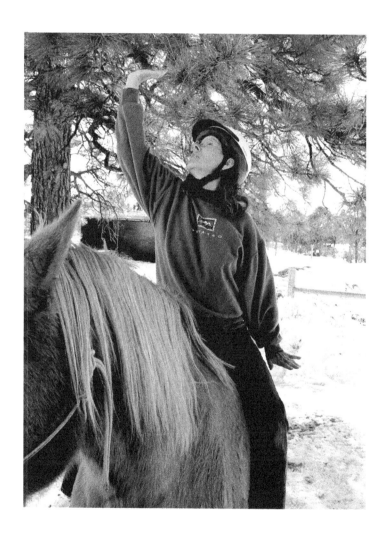

Raise your right arm and flatten your hand as if you are holding up the sky. Lower your left arm and flatten your hand as if you are holding down the earth. Look at the upward arm. Feel the stretch. Take several breaths and then repeat with the left arm raised, and the right arm down. Again, look at the upward arm. This pose strengthens the shoulders and the back muscles.

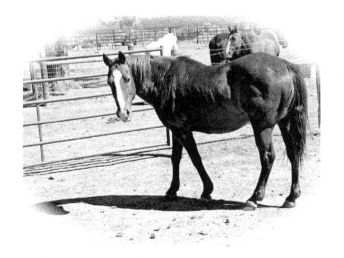

Now for something different! Do the next twelve poses in a flowing sequence one right after the other like a dance. This group of poses relieves tension and enhances circulation.

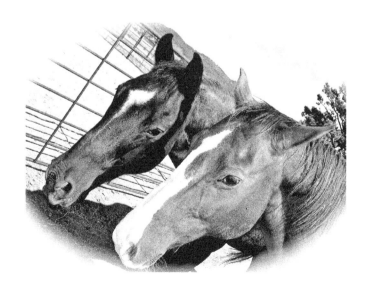

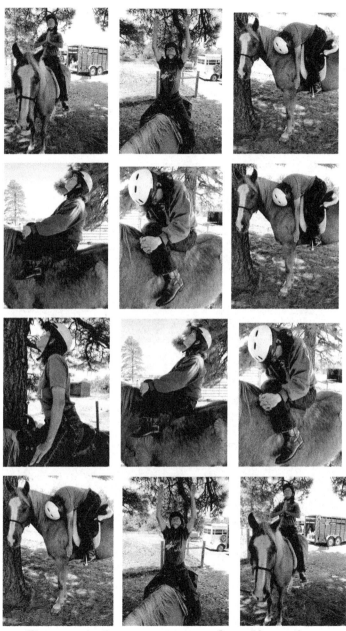

Turn to the next page for directions.

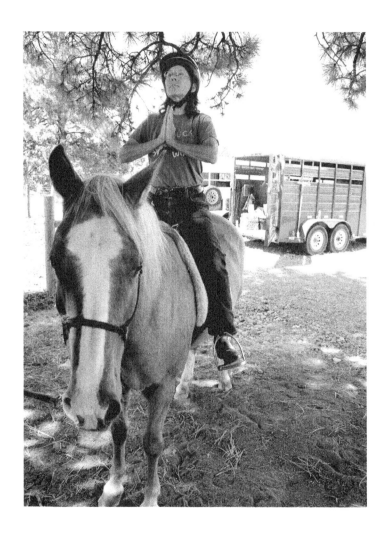

Hands to your heart, with palms together.

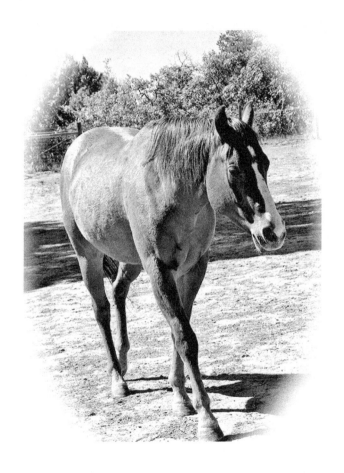

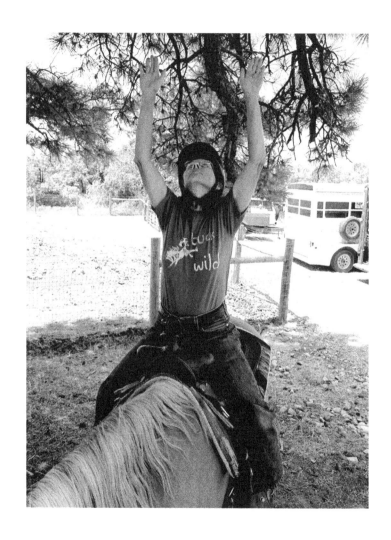

Inhale and reach upward with your arms, looking up, and arching your back.

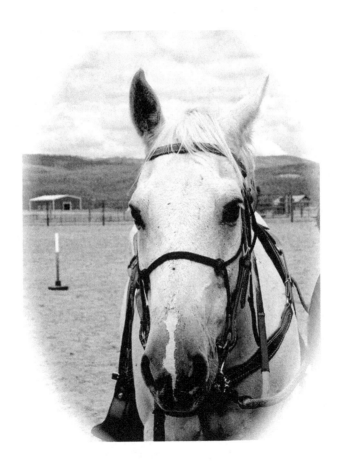

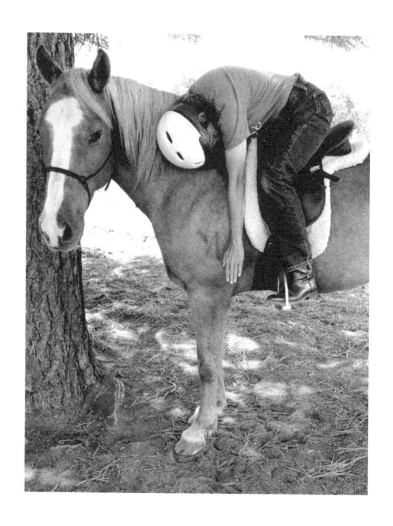

Exhale, and bend forward slowly, with your hands beside your feet.

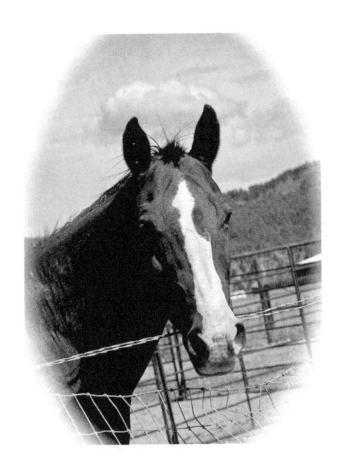

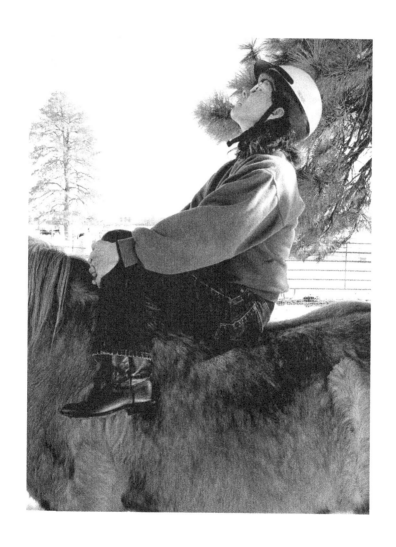

Inhale, and pull your left knee into
your chest. Look upward, and
have your back slightly arched.

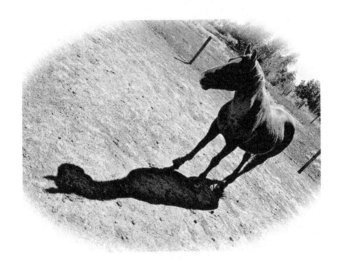

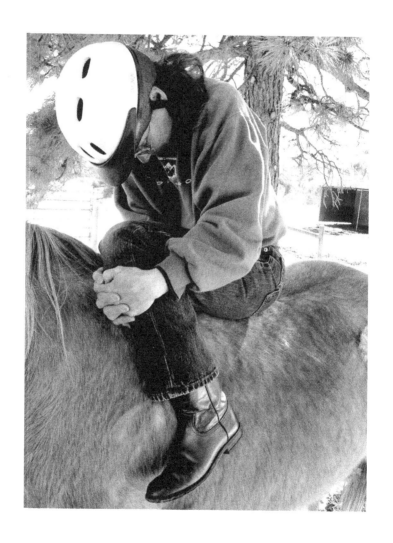

Start to exhale as you bring your chin to your chest and your forehead to your knee.

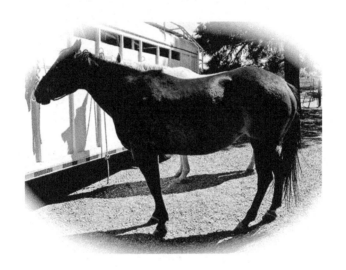

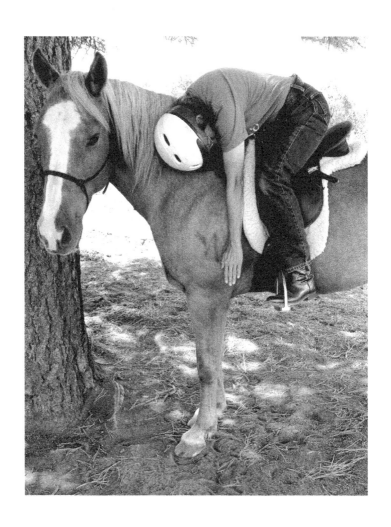

Finish your exhale as you bend forward slowly, with your hands beside your feet.

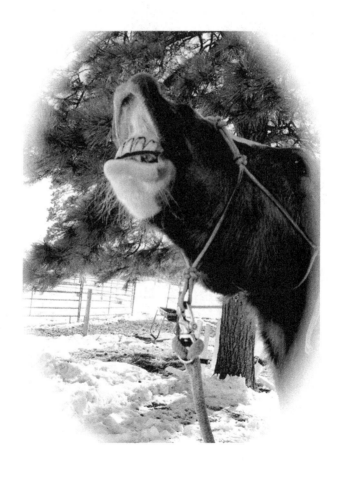

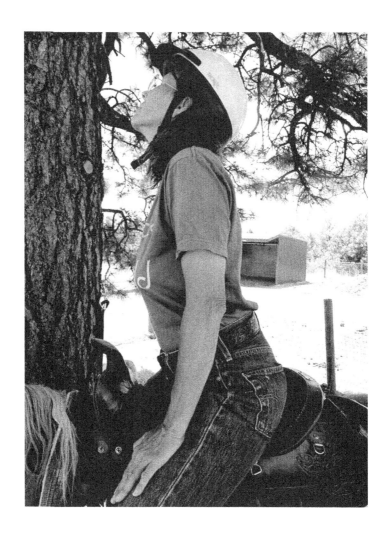

Start to inhale as you arch your back and neck, with your hands down by your legs.

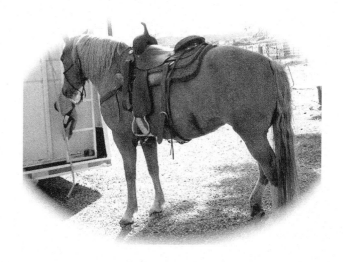

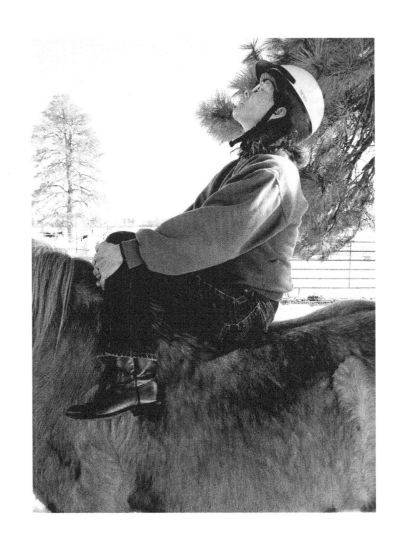

Complete your inhale as you pull your right knee toward your chest. Look upward and have your back slightly arched.

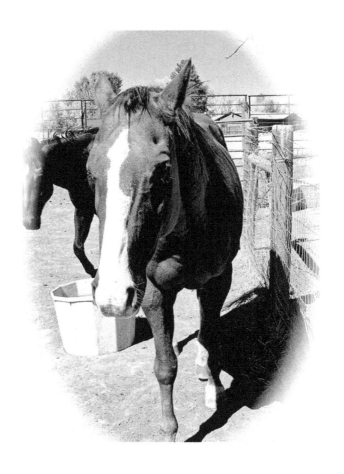

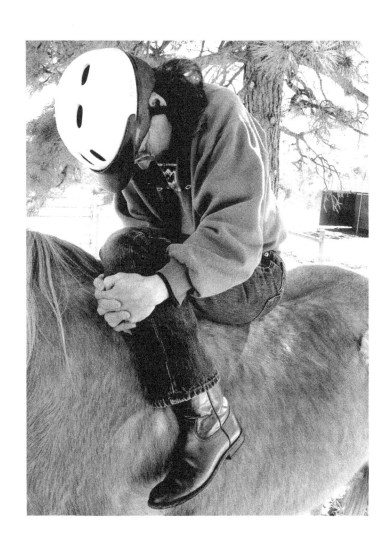

Start to exhale as you bring your chin to your chest and your forehead toward your knee.

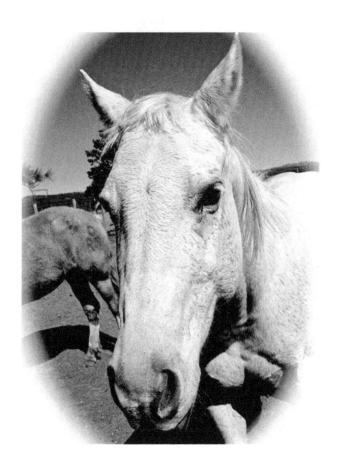

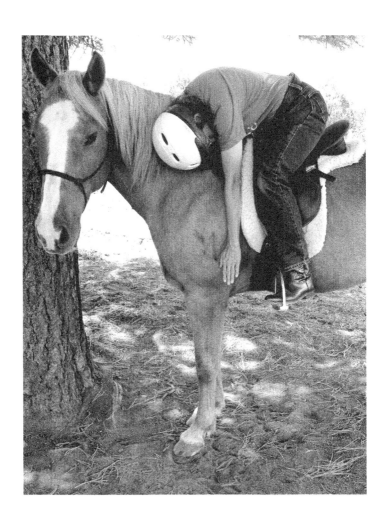

Finish your exhale as you bend forward slowly, with your hands beside your feet.

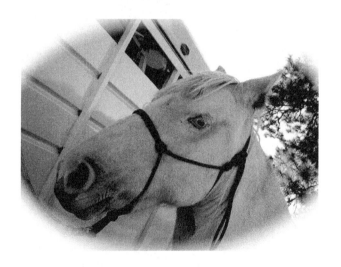

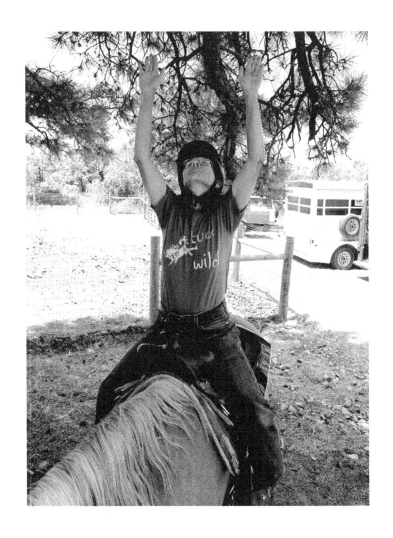

Inhale and reach upward with your arms, looking up, and arching your back.

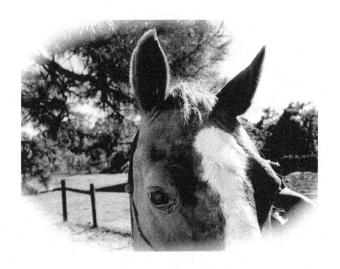

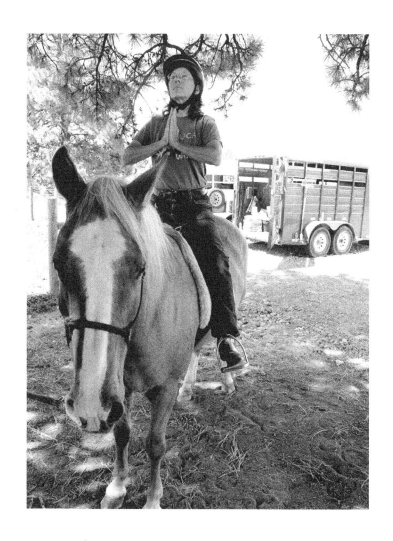

Exhale. Hands to your heart, with palms together.

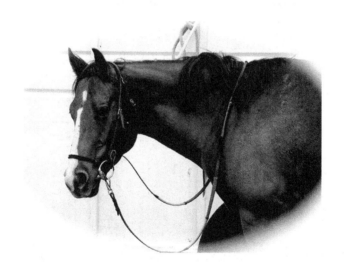

The End

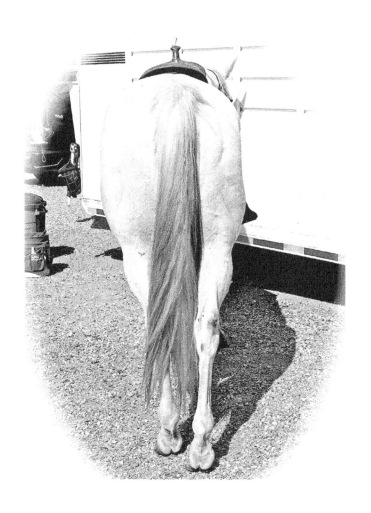

Made in the USA
Monee, IL
01 April 2022

93955665R00059